MY PREGNANCY CARE WITH GESTATIONAL DIABETES: TIPS ON DIET, GROCERY SHOPPING AND EATING OUT

BY MATHEA FORD, RDN, LD

PURPOSE AND INTRODUCTION

What I have found through the emails and requests of my readers is that it is difficult to find information about a gestational diabetes program that is actionable. I want you to know that is what I intend to provide in all my books. You can take this information from the book and with immediate action you will have a better outcome in your life.

I wrote this module with you in mind: the mom to be with gestational diabetes who does not know where to start or can't seem to get the answers that you need from other sources. This book will provide information that is applicable to a gestational diabetes mom.

Who am I? I am a registered dietitian in the USA who has been working with kidney patients for my entire 15 + years of experience. I was also in your shoes, as a mom to be with gestational diabetes (and now 2 children who are 7 &9) Find all my books on Amazon on my author page: http://www.amazon.com/Mathea-Ford/e/B008E1E7IS/

My goals are simple – to give some answers and to create an understanding of what is typical. In this series for Baby Steps For Gestational Diabetes, I will take you through the different parts of being a woman with gestational diabetes. It will not necessarily be what happens in your case, as everyone is an individual. I may simplify things in an effort to write them so that I feel you can learn the most from the information. This may mean that I don't say the exact things that your doctor would say. If you don't understand, please ask your doctor.

I want you to know, I am not a medical doctor and I am not aware of your particular condition. Information in this book is current as of publication, but may or may not have changed.

This book is not meant to substitute for medical treatment for you, your friends, your caregivers, or your family members. You should not base treatment decisions solely on what is contained in this module. Develop your treatment plan with your doctors, nurses and the other medical professionals on your team. I recommend that you double-check any information with your medical team to verify if it applies to you.

In other words, I am not responsible for your medical care. I am providing this module for information and entertainment purposes, not medical diagnoses. Please consult with your doctor about any questions that you have about your particular case.

We do understand that babies are both male and female, but in the interest of making sure that you can clearly distinguish mom we refer to the baby as he.

TABLE OF CONTENTS

WHAT IS GESTATIONAL DIABETES?

INTRODUCTION

Who doesn't want a healthy pregnancy and do what's best for their baby? That's why it is so important to go to your scheduled appointments with your doctor. They know how to help you through your pregnancy and can identify anything that may be amiss. Many pregnant women are not familiar with the many tests and procedures required in their pregnancy, especially when they are first time mothers. In your second trimester around weeks 24-28, one of the things they will test for is *gestational diabetes (GD)*.

Gestational diabetes is a kind of diabetes that happens during pregnancy. According to the March of Dines, four out of every 100 pregnant women develop gestational diabetes. Gestational diabetes is defined as "diabetes diagnosed during pregnancy that is not clearly overt diabetes," according to the American Diabetes Association. The word "gestational" refers to the time a baby is developing in a mother. *Diabetes* is a disease that means "too much sugar in the blood." The body cannot use the sugars and starches (carbohydrates) it takes in as food into the cells to make energy. The body either makes no insulin, too little insulin, or cannot use the insulin it makes to change those sugars and starches into energy. As a result, extra sugar builds up in the blood. More times than not, GD will resolve on its own after the birth of the baby. However, a mother's risk to develop diabetes in the next 5 to 10 years is increased. Gestational diabetes is on the rise in the US as the general population is increasing in weight and a higher proportion of the population becomes more obese.

Diabetes is often diagnosed in women during their childbearing years and can affect the health of both the mother and her unborn child. Poor control of diabetes during pregnancy increases the chances for birth defects and other problems for the baby. It can cause serious complications for the mom, also. Proper health care before and during pregnancy can help prevent birth defects and other poor outcomes according to the Centers for Disease Control.

RISK FACTORS FOR GESTATIONAL DIABETES

Risk factors are things that increase the likelihood that a person will obtain a certain disease. The risk factors for GD are obesity, family genetics or personal health history, age, and ethnicity.

OVERWEIGHT:

One thing that you should know is your body mass index or your BMI. BMI is the measure of your height to weight and is used by doctors as a measure of obesity. The more you weigh relative to how tall you are, the higher your BMI will be. You're more likely to develop gestational diabetes if you're significantly overweight with a body mass index (BMI) of 30 or higher. An article by MJ Evans, Diabetes and Pregnancy (2009), suggests that obese women are three times more likely to develop gestational diabetes than women whose BMI is in the healthy range. Many online calculators can help you figure out your BMI.

To get an idea of what weight is a normal weight for a woman who is 5'4", she should weigh between 110-140 pounds. Here the BMI range would be in the normal zone at 18.5 to 25. However, if her weight reaches 175 pounds or more, her BMI will be at 30, which is not good. This is where health problems are more likely to occur, such as diabetes and heart disease.

FAMILY OR PERSONAL HEALTH HISTORY:
If you have pre-diabetes or you have a close family member like your parents or siblings, that has type 2 diabetes, you will have an increased chance of GD. The chances increase if you had gestational diabetes with a prior pregnancy or you delivered a baby of more than 9 pounds. An unexplained stillbirth could also be a risk factor for GD. This means you should discuss with your doctor any need for early testing.

AGE GREATER THAN 25:
If you are older than 25 years of age during your pregnancy, you will have a higher chance of developing GD.

NON-CAUCASIAN:
If you are black, Hispanic, American Indian or Asian, you will be more likely to develop gestational diabetes.

CAUSES OF GESTATIONAL DIABETES
Hormones play a big part in why some women develop gestational diabetes. When a woman is pregnant, she produces hormones to sustain the growing fetus inside her womb. In some women, these hormones make the body's cells less responsive to insulin. The pancreas is the organ in the human body that secretes *insulin* when there is glucose (or sugar) in the blood. Think of insulin as the gatekeeper to our cells. Glucose floats around freely in our blood, but it is needed to provide energy for the cells. This is where insulin comes in. Insulin attaches itself to cells allowing the glucose to enter our hungry cells. The cells, in turn, can use the glucose for energy and do their functions.

When the pregnancy hormones wreak havoc in the pregnant woman's body, the insulin may become less responsive and will not "open the door" to the cell for glucose to enter. The cells will not get the needed glucose and will not function properly. The pancreas will sense there is too much glucose in the blood stream and will respond by working harder putting out more insulin. This response does not help to improve insulin sensitivity, however. Excess blood glucose in the body will continue unless controlled by diet, exercise, and/or medication.

WHY BOTHER WORRYING ABOUT HIGH BLOOD SUGAR?

Are you thinking about ignoring your doctor's advice since you feel like your sugar is just a "little" high? You should understand the implications of not controlling your blood sugar. First of all, when you continue to eat as you wish, you are causing yourself to gain more weight and increase your chances for a C-section. The baby gets too much sugar from you and becomes larger than normal. Additionally, you are increasing your chances in developing overt diabetes in the long term. This is the cycle that will lead you to feel bad and worsen your diabetes.

Gestational diabetes may also increase the mother's risk of:

HIGH BLOOD PRESSURE, PREECLAMPSIA AND ECLAMPSIA

The risk for developing high blood pressure increases with GD. It will also raise your risk for preeclampsia and eclampsia. These are two very serious complications that can be dangerous for both the baby and the mother. It decreases the blood circulation to the baby and the mother could go into a seizure. Pre-eclampsia is a condition in which a mom develops high blood pressure, retains too much fluid and damages her kidneys.

FUTURE DIABETES

If you develop GD, you are more likely to develop it again in any future pregnancies. Also you are more likely to develop type 2 diabetes when you get older. You can avoid this by controlling your blood glucose, eating better, exercising regularly, and maintaining a healthy weight.

EFFECTS ON THE BABY

As far as her baby, he could develop complications including macrosomia (a baby that weighs more than 9 pounds), neonatal hypoglycemia (low blood sugar), respiratory distress syndrome (trouble breathing), shoulder displacement, polycythemia (excess blood cells), and hypocalcaemia (low calcium) (Setji et al., 2005).

EXCESSIVE BIRTH WEIGHT

When a mom to be eats too many carbohydrates, this causes extra glucose to go to the baby in the womb. The umbilical cord carries blood and nutrients from the mother so any extra nutrients are provided to the fetus. Excess sugar to the baby makes him gain weight quicker than he should. An overweight baby is at risk for injury upon delivery. This includes injury to the shoulder, injury to the nerves in his neck, fractured collarbone or lack of oxygen. Because of this, the baby will more likely be taken by C-section, which poses its own risks.

EARLY (PRETERM) BIRTH AND RESPIRATORY DISTRESS SYNDROME

There is a chance that if the mother does not keep her blood sugar under control, her high blood sugar will increase her chances of going into premature labor and putting the baby at risk. A complication of a baby with a mother with gestational diabetes could be respiratory distress syndrome. Babies with this have difficulty breathing because their lungs are not fully developed. They will need help breathing until their lungs develop more. Even if a baby of a mother with gestational diabetes is not premature, it still has the risk of respiratory distress syndrome. Moms with large babies are more likely to have a c-section for delivery.

LOW BLOOD SUGAR (HYPOGLYCEMIA)
There is a risk that a baby could have low blood sugar (hypoglycemia) shortly after birth because he has just come from having excess glucose pumped in its bloodstream from its mother and its pancreas is still pumping high amounts of insulin out. The baby could experience seizures because of low blood sugars once the source of glucose is removed (the connection with the mom through the umbilical cord), so feedings need to start immediately and possibly an IV of glucose solution to bring the baby's blood sugar back to normal.

SHOULDER DYSTOCIA OR BIRTH INJURY
Because of the increased weight of the baby, there is more of a chance that the baby will suffer injury upon birth through the birth canal.

CAESAREAN DELIVERY
Because of the risk of a large baby passing through the birth canal, a C-section may be warranted. Additionally, if there are complications with the pregnancy, the physician will want to take the baby early if it is in a compromising position.

JAUNDICE
Jaundice is possible because the baby's liver isn't mature enough to breakdown its bilirubin, which are old or damaged red blood cells that the body is trying to remove. The baby's skin and whites of its eye will be a yellowish tone. Jaundice is not a major concern but needs to be monitored. The baby may be put through light therapy to help rid him of the jaundice.

Coincidently, babies are at higher risk of type 2 diabetes in mothers with GD and may become obese in their lifetime.

Close Monitoring Of The Baby

A woman whose blood glucose levels are not controlled or require insulin therapy, have high blood pressure, or a history of stillbirth will receive more intensive fetal monitoring. The baby will be affected by high blood sugar in the mother so he will be closely monitored by the following assessments and tests:

a. **Non-stress test**. The Non-stress test (NST) is a non-invasive test performed in pregnancies 28 weeks or more. It is done at the doctor's office and will take about ½ an hour to do. The mother is laid on her back on the exam table and asked to relax.
A belt will be wrapped around the mother's abdomen to detect the fetus' heart beat and another belt will be used to monitor contractions. The whole point of the test is to measure the baby's heart rate when it's moving in the womb. If the baby is active, its heart rate should increase. The idea is to see if the fetus is getting enough oxygen. If the baby is active but the heart rate is slow, it may not be getting the oxygen needed.

b. **Biophysical profile (BPP)**. A biophysical profile (BPP) test is used to keep track of the baby's health. Ultrasound methods are used to track various things such as heart rate, muscle tone, rate of breathing, and the amount of amniotic fluid.

c. **Fetal movement counting.** The physician will like to see the fetus movement at around 10 movements in a two-hour period. Many times moms are asked to track this over a couple of days every week.

At the time of labor and having the baby, the blood glucose of the mother will be monitored every 2 hours so the level of 100 mg/dl or less is maintained as well as the baby's blood sugar level. This is to decrease the risk of the baby having hypoglycemia after birth and to ensure the mother's blood sugars return to normal after delivery.

TREATMENTS AND MEDICATIONS

The physician or dietitian will discuss with you about blood sugars and how to recognize high and low blood sugar. Also they will tell you what they mean and how to manage them.

HIGH BLOOD SUGAR

Your doctor should let you know what guidelines to follow while monitoring your blood sugar at home. If your blood sugar after fasting (most likely when you get up in the morning before you eat anything) is at or above 106 mg/dl or above, it is too high. Anything at 153 mg/dl or above two hours after you eat is considered a high blood sugar as well. If you find you are have a high glucose reading when you check it at home, you can counter this by exercising more (a simple 10 minute walk would do). You may also need to review what you ate to see if there is a food that is causing your blood sugar to spike. Skipping meals or snacks may cause the body to compensate and release more blood glucose producing a high reading, so do not skip any meals or snacks!

LOW BLOOD SUGAR

Low blood sugar is a concern, too. A reading under 70 mg/dl means you need to take in some quick carbohydrates. Hypoglycemia, or low blood sugar, is more common if you are taking the oral medication, glyburide, or you are taking insulin shots. It can occur because you didn't eat enough to make up for the insulin you took or exercised more than normal. Hypoglycemia can happen anytime. You may feel woozy or "just not right" before your scheduled blood sugar check. Go ahead and check it early anyway. If it is low, drink something sweet like orange juice (about 4 ounces or 15 grams of carbohydrate) or eat some candy. A sweet beverage will act quicker on your blood sugar. You should check your blood glucose again in fifteen minutes to ensure that it is up to an acceptable level (over 90 mg/dl but under 140 mg/dl). It is important to maintain optimal blood sugar levels for you and the health of the baby.

MONITORING YOUR BLOOD SUGAR

Some good reference information for blood sugar levels are shown in this table:

TIMING OF BLOOD SUGAR	NORMAL RANGE (mg/dl)
When you wake (before eating)	80 to 105
Before eating a meal	80 to 120
Taken 2 hours after eating	Less than 140
Bedtime blood sugar range	100 to 140

(http://bloodsugarlevelsnormal.com/blood-sugar-chart-what-do-the-numbers-mean/)

The goal for therapy in GD is strict blood glucose control. The fasting blood glucose should be less than 105 mg/dl and 2-hour after meal blood levels should be less than 120 mg/dl. Your doctor's expected blood level values may be a little different, so be sure to ask.

Your physician will possibly refer you to a dietitian, a health professional who is well-trained in diabetic counseling. They will introduce you to a piece of equipment called a *glucometer*. This is a small machine that will read your blood sugar level.

HEALTHY DIET

Dietary modification is the number one intervention in the treatment of GD. The basic prescription for the diet will equate to around 2000 to 2400 calories a day. You are not restricted in what you have, but you need to watch the carb count that is allotted for each meal and snack. If you go over the recommended carbs, your blood sugar will be high. In chapter 2, dietary meals and carb counting will be discussed. The dietitian will encourage you to opt for more healthy choices such as fruits and vegetables over eating muffins and other sweets.

EXERCISE

Exercise is a wonderful way to control your diabetes. It burns calories as well as any sugar in the blood that would otherwise be causing problems. Exercise doesn't have to be vigorous to be effective. It is best done after meals, when blood glucose is the highest. It is important to self-monitor blood glucose levels before, during, and after exercise to determine the effect exercise has on your blood sugar level. Be on the alert after you exercise that you don't experience hypoglycemia, or low blood sugar, which may occur up to several hours after the activity. Walking is a great activity to do every day since you can do it about anywhere and it is easy to do. Consider swimming if you have access to the local Y or community pool. Swimming is a low-impact exercise that gets your whole body moving. Any activity you enjoy doing will help in controlling gestational diabetes.

So how do you get started with exercise? Try to pick an activity that you enjoy. If you do this, you will be more likely to stick with it for the long term. You want to find one that fits into your lifestyle. Things to consider would be your normal routine, access to the equipment needed, and any costs, like a membership to the health club. You need to have a good pair of shoes and socks as part of your exercise routine.

Next, consider doing some goal setting for the next couple of months. Write your goals down on a calendar or in a journal. You may not want to do a full-fledged exercise program, but you can aim to increase your activity in some way. First, think of what type of exercise you will do. Next, decide how often. You will need to be specific like "three times a week" or "every other day." How long will you exercise? Again, be specific. Altogether, it will look similar to this statement: "I will walk for 30 minutes every day after dinner." It defines the "what," "when" and "how often" in your exercise goal. You can always re-evaluate your goals if you find you need to decrease and increase your exercise. Ultimately, try not to overdo it. You may only need to work out 20 minutes a day to control your blood sugars.

It helps to keep track of your goals when you start an exercise program. Have a journal or calendar to mark for each day you meet your target goal. Your dietitian may give you a log book where you can fill in your activity for each day as well. You will feel a sense of accomplishment when you see that you finished each day with a check mark or the minutes you completed. You can use a pedometer when you walk to measure the steps. That would be another great way to measure your progress. Just remember, no one is perfect. If you miss a day, you just start up the next day.

When you are exercising, always keep hydrated. This is important, especially if you have GD, because dehydration can cause your blood sugar to go up (Toiba, 2013). Even if you do not feel thirsty, you need to drink fluids before, during, and after exercise. How much do you need to drink?

Before exercise: 8 ounces of water

During exercise: 8 ounces for every 20 minutes (more if you sweat a lot; drink this while you exercise)

After exercise: 8 ounces or more

Warm-up is recommended with your daily exercise regimen. This helps start your activity with a gradual increase in heart rate at the beginning of the activity. To do this, you can do a casual walk for a few minutes and then do some stretches to warm up the muscles. Cool-down after exercise is just as important to help your heart rate ease down. Warm-up and cool-down are especially important if you haven't exercised in a while.

Take your blood sugar reading before and after exercise if you are on insulin therapy. You will need to take a snack in case you begin to feel faint. Carry a cell phone with you and have the emergency number on your contact list as ICE: in case of emergency. You might even find a partner who enjoys exercising with you, just make sure they are a motivated as you to exercise or you might find it tough to go.

MEDICATION

There are several types of medications that the doctor may prescribe if you cannot control your blood sugar by diet and exercise alone. The doctor may start by prescribing an oral medication. A patient with GD will still need to watch their diet and blood sugars. Dietary change may be the first-line management, but oral medication should be quickly instituted if sufficient response is not obtained. Fast-acting insulin along with slower-acting insulin will be the treatment utilized if oral medication doesn't do the trick. The doctor will adjust the dosages as the pregnancy progresses as insulin resistance seems to increase as time goes on.

Remember it's for the health of your baby. You are not a "failure" if you need insulin. Your body just needs some adjustments and help, and you are doing what you need to do to have a healthy baby.

Metformin

Metformin is a common oral diabetic medication, although not officially licensed for use during pregnancy, it has gained acceptance as the optional treatment for GD and is recommended by the National Institute for Health and Care Excellence, Metformin appears to be both safe and effective, with the risk of perinatal complications being no higher than in insulin-treated patients" The metformin therapy shows that insulin requirements and weight gain are lower. After birth, medication is usually withdrawn in gestational diabetes and blood glucose levels monitored to see if the mother's own insulin production goes back to normal.

Insulin

If the oral medication is not controlling the blood sugars, insulin may need to be prescribed. The American College of Obstetricians and Gynecologists recommends that women who continuously hit the thresholds of 105 mg/dl fasting blood sugar and 120 mg/dl blood sugars after meals need to start on insulin therapy. Insulin is the pharmacological choice in all women with diabetes during pregnancy. Insulin is a natural part of the body so it will not affect the baby in a harmful way. Insulin is started at a low dose and increased weekly until the desired blood sugar range is obtained. When insulin is given, it is injected directly into the fatty tissue, usually with a little syringe. The needle is much smaller than the one used to give a flu shot. It is given in the abdomen or thigh. The doses may need to be increased the remainder of the pregnancy since the mother's insulin resistance will rise as well. In addition to self-monitoring of blood glucose, a lab draw called the A1c will be taken every 2 to 4 weeks, aiming for the value of <6%. GD women can stop insulin after the delivery of the baby and placenta as long as lab test indicate they are in the normal range. You will be giving yourself the insulin shots every day and you will have to learn to do it yourself. At first, this might be difficult. Once you do it a few times, it gets easier. Your doctor or diabetes educator will help you with the technique.

Breastfeeding

Most doctors will recommend that you breast-feed, if possible, for the health benefits for you and your baby. For example, breast-feeding can help keep your child at a healthy weight, which may reduce his or her chances of developing diabetes. It provides antibodies to strengthen your baby's immune system, and it lowers your baby's risk for many types of infections. And it may lower your chances of developing diabetes later in life.

UNDERSTANDING THE FOODS YOU EAT

The dietitian you meet with will discuss with you the different types of nutrients you need to be aware of when planning your diet. The main ones will be carbohydrates, protein, and fats.

CARBOHYDRATES:

Carbohydrates are a major part of our lives when it comes to eating. Sugar, flour, and anything made with them is a carbohydrate. Fruit and vegetables are carbohydrates as well as anything from the grain group such as rice, oatmeal, and wheat; milk is very important especially with pregnancy. All carbohydrates contain 4 calories per gram. Complex carbohydrates are carbs in their most natural form, like whole grain and fresh vegetables. These types of carbohydrates are preferred over simple carbohydrates because they absorb more slowly into the bloodstream, preventing blood sugar spikes. Starches can be refined or complex carbohydrates. They include certain vegetables, legumes, grains, and products made from grain, for instance, pasta.

Carbohydrates will be your main focus when it comes to watching what you eat for the remainder of your pregnancy. This is because carbohydrates are what influences your blood sugar. There are some carbohydrates which are better than others in how they are broken down by the body and work to raise blood sugar levels. Carbohydrate portions are recommended to be distributed over three meals and two to three snacks to minimize after meal high blood sugar spikes. Let's take a look at the different carbs we eat:

Refined Carbohydrates:

Refined carbohydrates are broken down quickly and easily digested, such as cakes and cookies. They are foods we eat that are processed. The more processed the food, the more refined. Here are some examples:

Sweetened Cereal, like Captain Crunch	Candy
	Pies
Cake	Pasta
Regular Cereal, like Cheerios	Bread
Cookies	

Refined carbohydrates are the ones that raise blood sugar rapidly. It doesn't take much for the digestive enzymes in your body to break this type of carb down into glucose and quickly send it into the blood stream. Essentially, it is dumping the sugar into your body all at once and overloading your body, and overwhelming your pancreas. Eating refined carbohydrates makes it difficult to control blood glucose levels. A serving of carbohydrate equals 15 grams of total carbohydrate as listed on the label.

Complex Carbohydrates
The best choice for you is eating complex carbohydrates. This type of carb is one that is as close to nature as you can get. We're talking vegetables straight out of the garden. Included in the list are also fruit and whole grains. These carbs are also full of fiber, which makes them slower to be broken down by the body's digestive system.

Complex carbohydrates are also full of the nutrients we need so that makes them the better choice. For blood sugar regulation, consuming complex carbs offers a slower release of glucose into the blood stream. This helps in preventing extreme highs and drops in blood sugar.

Glycemic Index

There is a measurement called the glycemic index (GI) that bases carbohydrates on a number scale by how fast they raise blood sugar and insulin in the body. The way the food gets assigned a GI number is how much of an increase of glucose it causes compared to pure glucose which is 100. For example, a food of a GI of 45 means it only boosts blood sugar by 45% as much as glucose. The lower the rating on this chart for a certain food, the better it is in terms of slow release of sugar into the bloodstream. For example, white bread is a 73, so it is almost as bad as eating pure sugar, according to the chart. You will find most vegetables and beans lower in the list. The more fiber a food contains, the lower it will be in the list as well. Below are examples of some foods and where they are at in the glycemic index:

Low GI

(55 or less): Most beans and colorful vegetables, meats

Moderate GI

(56-69): White and sweet potatoes, white rice

High GI

(70 and up): donuts, bread, cakes

If you stay with the lower GI foods, you will be more successful in keeping your blood sugars regulated. You can find a handy calculator for the glycemic index of any food at http://www.glycemicindex.com/. You will find that eating lower GI foods will keep you satisfied longer and keep hunger at bay, as well as help with blood sugar control.

How much carbohydrate?

You will have an allotted amount of carbohydrate for your day. Your meal plan will help be your guide. The following is a basic guideline of how many carb choices you may have in your meal plan:

Breakfast: 30-45 grams

Lunch: 60-75 grams

Dinner: 60-75 grams

Morning snack: 15-30 grams

Afternoon snack: 15-30 grams

Evening snack: 15-30 grams

We will discuss *carbohydrate counting* more in depth in the next chapter. If your blood sugars continue to be high, you might need to reduce the amount of carbohydrate or increase your exercise. But many women also need to take insulin to help control their blood sugars with gestational diabetes

Protein

Meat, nuts, eggs... this is where you can find your protein. It is essential to eat protein as it is used to maintain muscle. A pregnant woman's diet should comprise of between 10%-35% of protein. Fish, lean meats, poultry, and beans are the best options to add to your diet to meet this need. So eat 2 - 3 servings a day: one serving equals 2-3 oz. cooked meat, poultry, or fish; 1/2 cup cooked beans; 2 medium eggs; or 2 tablespoons peanut butter.

Fats

Fat gets a bad rap but fats are essential in our diet. The type of fats is what matters. Monounsaturated fats are a much healthier choice. Olive oil and sunflower oil are good examples. You want to stay away from saturated fats. Saturated fats are in products that are solid at room temperature like butter and shortening. Food labels list the individual fats on the products they are in. Saturated fats should be limited to less than 10% of total calories. So if a food you want to eat has 100 calories and 2 grams of saturated fat, you would calculate the percentage of saturated fat by first multiplying 2 grams by 9 calories (how many calories in every gram of fat). You would then divide the answer "18" by 100 to get 18%.

2 grams of saturated fat x 9 calories = 18 calories

18 calories ÷ 100 total calories = 18% saturated fat (goal is less than 10%)

You should not include this food in your meal planning as it is too high in saturated fat.

Artificial Sweeteners

If you need to add a little sweetness to your beverage in the morning, artificial sweeteners are fine, just as long as they are used in moderation. For example, two cans of diet cola per day would safe during pregnancy. Ask your doctor if you have any questions about how much he/she recommends.

CARBOHYDRATE COUNTING AND LABEL READING

Carbohydrates in your diet will influence your blood sugars, so planning is essential to control your readings. You will learn how to count carbs and read labels so that you are able to plan meals accordingly.

Carbohydrate Counting

It is important that you learn about carb counting. It isn't hard to learn once you know the concept. You will be reading nutritional facts labels to calculate carb units at each meal and snack.

You will be a "label reading expert" by the time you are done with your pregnancy. However, it is great information to use even after you have your baby. Knowing exactly what you put in your mouth is important even when you're not having health issues. Since having gestational diabetes increases the risk of having type 2 diabetes in the future, you can be still be proactive and watch what you eat to help prevent further problems. Knowing how to read labels will be beneficial now and later.

O.K., let's read our first food label:

Serving Size 2 whole crackers *(31 g)*

Servings Per Carton about 13

Amount per serving

Calories 130

Total Fat 3g

     Saturated Fat 0g

Trans Fat 0g

Monounsaturated 0.5g

Cholesterol 0mg

Sodium 140mg

Total Carbohydrate 25g

Dietary Fiber 1g

Sugars 8g

It is important to note what the serving size is. If you don't, you may think a whole packet of food is one serving when it may be three. This label shows that two whole crackers is a serving, and there are 13 servings per box. The serving is shown to have 130 calories in it. As you move down the list, you will see the total carbohydrate to be 25 grams and there is one gram of fiber. That is a very important part of the puzzle and key to pay attention to on the label.

Check out the following chart. By looking at it, you will see that there are two columns. One shows "total carbohydrate grams" and the other is what we call "carbohydrate choices." There are 15 grams of carbohydrate in a carb choice when you are carbohydrate counting. Now, if you are allowed only one carb choice (or 15 grams of carb) for a snack, you wouldn't be able to eat this product. However, you could eat only ONE cracker, instead of two.

25 carbs/2 servings = 12.5 carbohydrates or 1 carb choice

Total Carbohydrate Grams	Carbohydrate Choices
0-5	0
6-10	½
11-20	1
21-25	1 ½
26-35	2
36-40	2 ½
41-50	3
51-55	3 ½
56-65	4
66-70	4 ½
71-80	5
81-85	5 ½
86-95	6

However, you may want to choose a complex carbohydrate such as an apple because you will get more to eat. The apple is low on the glycemic index and more nutritious.

Most foods will have the carb count listed on the label but at other times you could need to do a calculation. Your dietitian will recommend your meal plan have x number of carbohydrates or x number of carb units.

You will see by the chart that the more carbs there is in a food, you will start "losing" carb points. How? Let us look at the carb count table: You can see where 11-20 grams of carbohydrates equals one carb choice (or unit). Do you think if you eat 40 grams of carbs of a certain food, you get 2 carb choices? According to the chart, you would get 2 ½. So that ½ carb choice that could've gone to more food is lost on the item you chose. You can't combine all of your carbohydrates for the day or even a meal and apply it to this chart. You will calculate each food as its own carb count.

Let's practice another one:

The following label information is on some nutrition bars. As you can see, the serving size listed here is just one bar. There are twelve servings in the box. Let's take a look at the label and figure out how many carb units are contained.

Serving size 1 bar

Servings per Container 12

Amount per serving

Calories 80

Total Fat 5g

> *Saturated Fat 4.5g*

> *Trans Fat 0g*

Cholesterol 5mg

Sodium 30mg

Total Carbohydrate 9g

> *Dietary Fiber 2g*

Sugars 2g

Sugar Alcohol 3g

To count carbohydrates, look at three things:

Serving size

Number of servings per container

Grams of total carbohydrate per serving

Listed in this label are carbohydrates numbering at 9 grams. This lies between 6-10 on the carb unit chart and would count as ½ of a unit. You are allowed to subtract *half* the fiber (1 gram) and half the sugar alcohol (1.5 grams) here but it wouldn't make much of a significant difference. (Sugar alcohols are sometimes added to increase the sweetness but keep the sugar low. Too much of them can cause gastric distress) So this bar counts as ½ a carbohydrate serving. Let's take a look at another label.

Serving size ¾ cup

Servings per container 15

Amount per serving

Calories 100

Total Fat 0.5g

    Saturated Fat 0g

    Trans Fat 0g

Cholesterol 0mg

Sodium 220mg

Total Carbohydrate 24g

Dietary Fiber 6g

Sugars 5g

Sugar Alcohols 2g

The label above indicates one serving size (¾ cup) and contains 24 grams of carbohydrates. It shows it has 6 grams of dietary fiber and 2 sugar alcohols. In this example, you would see that 24 grams would convert to 1 1/2 carb choices (or units). However, you are allowed to subtract *half* the dietary fiber from the carbohydrate grams. So 24 grams minus 3 grams of dietary fiber brings the total to 21 grams. But wait! There are sugar alcohols to count as well. You do the same thing as with the dietary fiber. Take ½ of the sugar alcohol (1 gram) and subtract it from 21. You have a grand total of 20 grams of countable carbohydrates. If you look at the carb choice chart again, you will see that this product will be worth 1 carb choice.

6 grams of fiber/2 = 3 grams of countable fiber

2 grams of sugar alcohol= 1 gram of countable sugar alcohol

24 Total Carbohydrates – (3 grams of fiber + 1 gram of sugar alcohol) = 20 grams of countable carbohydrate

Let's try another one. Below is a food label for a serving of three cookies.

Serving size 3 cookies

Servings about 5

Amount per serving

Calories 160

Total Fat 9g

Saturated Fat 3.5g

Trans Fat 0g

Cholesterol less than 5mg

Sodium 130mg

Total Carbohydrate 20g

Dietary Fiber 1g

Sugars 0g

Sugar Alcohols 7g

The number of carbohydrates is 20 grams, while it contains 1 gram of dietary fiber and 7 grams of sugar alcohol. This means you are allowed to subtract half of the dietary fiber and half of the sugar alcohol. So by taking 20 grams of carbs and subtract 0.5 grams of fiber and 3.5 grams of sugar alcohol, you come up with 20-4=16. The three cookies will count as one carb choice.

Be careful with reading the boxes many products are contained in. They may say there are sugar-free but that does not mean they are carbohydrate-free. A sugar-free label means that one serving has less than 0.5 gram of sugar. That is why it is so important to read labels. We need to know how many carbohydrates are in a food before you eat it, not how much sugar is in it. Many labels can be misleading as well. You have to be careful to not assume that a package is a serving size. Look at this label:

Serving size ¼ cup

Servings per container about 14

Amount per serving

Calories 190

Total Fat 16g

   Saturated Fat 1.5g

Cholesterol 0mg

Sodium 0mg

Total Carbohydrate 8g

   Dietary Fiber 1g

   Sugars 0g

You may presume that you can have a cup of this product as a serving, but if you look at the label, a quarter of a cup is a serving size and is also one carb choice. If you ate a cup of this, you would have used up 3 ½ to 4 carb choices!

When you're choosing between standard products and their sugar-free counterparts, compare the food labels. If the sugar-free product has noticeably fewer carbohydrates, the sugar-free product might be the better choice. But if there's little difference in carbohydrate grams between the two foods, let taste — or price — be your guide. Remember, a label of "no sugar added" does not mean "no carbohydrates." Although these foods don't contain high-sugar ingredients and no sugar is added during processing or packaging, foods without added sugar may still be high in carbohydrates.

Once you get carb counting down, you will start to piece together your meal plan. You will need to know how to count your calories as prescribed by your doctor. If your food is packaged, all you need to do is read the label and add the calorie and carbohydrate totals.

Meal Planning for Gestational Diabetes

It is very important to create a meal plan so you know where to allot your carbohydrates throughout the day. It should be designed to place your carbs in fairly equal increments to prevent high sugar spikes. It is beneficial to plan 3 meals and 3 snacks so you feel full and energetic.

Eating protein and fiber with your carbohydrate choices will keep your blood sugar regulated much better as they will slow the release of glucose into your blood stream. The key is to keep the blood sugar constant, without dips and elevations in the readings.

How Many Calories Should I Eat?

Many women think that they need to follow a very strict diet with gestational diabetes so that they do not harm the baby. Your diet is critical to your weight gain and your health. But the most important part of the diet is not the calories overall but the carbohydrate portions you eat. You may find that you are able to eat more food but less carbohydrate. Eating healthy involves more fiber and modest portions.

Pregnancy is not a time to lose weight, though. It is a time for measured weight gain that is healthy. So, you are not going on a crash diet to lose weight, you are growing a healthy baby. Most moms to be eat about 2000 – 2400 calories on a gestational diabetes diet. When you break that up into a meal plan, it ends up being about 50 – 55% carbohydrate, 30% fat, and 15 – 20% protein.

For a 2000 calorie diet, that is about 250 grams of carbohydrate per day, and 60 per meal (3 meals per day) and 15 – 25 per snack (3 per day). In carbohydrate counting it's about 4 carbohydrate servings per meal.

For a 2400 calorie diet, that is about 300 gm of carbohydrate per day, and 75 per meal (3 meals per day) and 15 – 25 per snack (3 per day). In carbohydrate counting, it's about 5 carbohydrate servings per meal.

Of course, everyone is different. Your diet should be individualized and it will take some time to see how different foods affect your blood sugar. It is recommended to space meals and snacks evenly. High-fiber carbohydrates and 2 ounces of protein is a good snack at bedtime so that blood sugar will not elevate or dip during the night. You may be wondering how it would elevate when you are not eating? Your liver is the culprit in that phenomenon. If your blood sugar dips for too long, the liver will send glucose into your blood. Then you will see a high fasting blood glucose reading in the morning. Exercise in your daily routine will help this, but if not, then the doctor may prescribe an oral medication.

Having the meal plan made out a week at a time will help you create a grocery list of what you need to keep in the house. You can involve your family in the planning as well so that everyone can participate. This will increase their support for you during this time.

There are a couple of ways you can plan your meals. Each will be discussed in detail and you then can choose which one works best for you.

CHOOSE YOUR PLATE

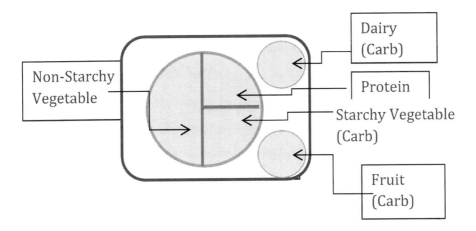

The "Choose Your Plate" plan doesn't count carbohydrates as it is more like portion control instead of strict counts. Basically load your plate up with low-carb vegetables first and you won't overdo it on the starchy carbs. Low-carb vegetables may include:

Cabbage	Bamboo Shoots	Mushrooms
Broccoli	Cucumbers	Okra
Carrots	Green Beans	Parsnips
Brussels Sprouts	Onions	Spinach
Tomatoes	Peppers	Summer Squash
Asparagus	Celery	Spaghetti Squash
Lettuce (all varieties)	Kohlrabi	
	Leeks	Cauliflower
Artichoke Hearts	Collard Greens	Radishes

Sauerkraut	Water Chestnuts
Rutabagas	Zucchini

Many people are visual learners and the diagram above really illustrates nicely how your plate should look when balancing your carbohydrates, protein, and fats. This simple method helps you to visualize the amount of vegetables, starch, and meat that should fill a 9-inch plate. For lunch and dinner half of the plate is filled with low-carb vegetables. Then one fourth is meat (2-3 ounces) and the other fourth is a starch. One glass of low-fat milk is included as well as a piece of fruit. The breakfast plate is ½ protein and ¼ optional starch. Low-fat milk completes the breakfast. This method is easy for a lot of people who do not want to do calculations but still keep their carbohydrates under control.

The following is an example:

First thing to do is fill your plate with the non-starchy vegetables. This can be the lettuce for your salad, green beans, sliced tomatoes, anything that is low-carb. This way you are not filling up your plate the majority of your plate with high carb foods. If you use half of your plate for the lower carb vegetables, you are doing great! Then you fill a quarter of it with starchy vegetables or whole-grain pasta. The remainder will be for your protein, such as chicken, fish, or beef. Add a serving of low-fat milk and a fruit serving, and you have your complete meal! This is an easy way to control your portions without the hassle of measuring out food. With this method, you end up with about 45-60 grams of carbohydrate at a meal. You can visit www.ChooseMyPlate.gov for more information on this technique of watching your food intake.

MEAL PLANNING WITH CARBOHYDRATE COUNTING

Now that you know how to count carbs, you may find you prefer this way of meal planning. The following is a general guideline of how your dietitian may have your carbohydrates distributed throughout the day. The other food groups are included as well. Remember, fiber and protein help slow the release of glucose into your body, keeping blood sugar levels stable. Milk should be included in the carb count, and you should drink one serving at lunch and dinner to help meet your calcium needs. Do not drink milk or fruit juice at breakfast as they tend to cause an increase in after breakfast blood sugars. Remember 15 grams of carbohydrate = 1 carbohydrate choice, so reading labels is very helpful.

Breakfast
2-3 Carbohydrate Choices (no fruit or juice at breakfast)

1 Serving of Protein

1 Serving of Fat (1 Tbsp butter or oil (45 calories))

Mid-morning snack
1-2 Carbohydrate Choice

1 Serving of Protein

Lunch
4-5 Carbohydrates Choices

Unlimited Non-Starch Vegetables

1 Serving of Protein (3 ounces of lean/medium meat)

1 Serving of Fat (1 Tbsp butter or oil (45 calories))

Mid-afternoon snack
1-2 Carbohydrate Choice

Dinner
4-5 Carbohydrates Choices

Unlimited Non-Starch Vegetables

1 Serving of Protein (3 ounces of lean/medium meat)

1 Serving of Fat (1 Tbsp butter or oil (45 calories))

Evening Snack
1 Carbohydrate Choice

1 Serving of Protein

Here is a sample seven-day meal plan to give you an idea of how your meals should look.

Day 1
Breakfast

Oatmeal, eggs, and water

Snack

Grapes and cheese slices

Lunch

Tuna salad, crackers, celery, grapes, and milk

Snack

Orange and cottage cheese

Dinner

Beef stew, sweet potatoes, green beans, apple, and milk

Snack
1 Slice whole grain bread

1 ounce cheese slice

Day 2

Breakfast

Eggs, light toast, and no-carb beverage

Snack

Apples with cheese slices

Lunch

Chicken with 2 slices light bread, steamed cauliflower, canned fruit in juice, and milk

Snack

Apricots and yogurt

Dinner

Grilled tilapia, broccoli, potato wedges, and milk

Snack
1 piece fruit

1 ounce cheese slice

Day 3

Breakfast

Small banana, Canadian bacon, and coffee

Snack

Melon and crackers

Lunch

Tortilla wrap with chicken, lettuce, and tomatoes, pear, and milk

Snack

Celery sticks and peanut butter

Dinner

Beef roast, salad, carrots, asparagus, canned fruit in juice, and milk

Snack
1 Slice whole grain bread
1 ounce deli meat

Day 4

Breakfast

Oatmeal with flax seed and coffee

Snack

Apple and peanuts

Lunch

Sandwich on light bread with ham/cheese and romaine lettuce, orange, and milk

Snack

Salad and hard-boiled egg

Dinner

Beef stir fry with broccoli and water chestnuts, brown rice, salad, fresh fruit, and milk

Snack
1 pear

1 ounce peanut butter

Day 5
Breakfast

Oatmeal, cantaloupe, and beverage

Snack

Salad with sunflower seeds

Lunch

Hamburger patty with low-carb bun, lettuce, tomato, peas, fresh fruit, and milk

Snack

Carrots and crackers

Dinner

Baked chicken, acorn squash, green beans, fresh fruit, and milk

Snack
¼ cup nuts

1 ounce of cheese

Day 6
Breakfast

Apple; mini muffin; coffee

Snack

Small baked potato with cheese

Lunch

Ground beef, cheese, salsa on low-carb tortilla shell, corn, and milk

Snack

Smoothie with yogurt and strawberries

Dinner

Beef roast, salad, green beans, fresh fruit, and milk

Snack

¾ cup milk

¾ cup high fiber cereal

Day 7
Breakfast

Cereal, apple, and unsweetened coffee (or with artificial sweetener)

Snack

Crackers with cheese

Lunch

Tomato soup, grilled cheese with whole wheat bread, grapes, and milk

Snack

Peaches and cottage cheese

Dinner

Spaghetti with sauce; lettuce salad with cucumbers, fresh fruit, and milk

Snack
6 Graham cracker squares

1 ounce nut butter

SIMPLE THINGS TO REMEMBER
When planning your meals, keep the following in mind. Though milk is an important part of your diet, drink it throughout the day rather than all at once. It is a liquid form of carbohydrate so

drinking it in one setting will cause your blood sugar to elevate quickly. Fruit is also important but too much will also affect your glucose readings. It has natural sugar in it so if you want it, be sure to eat it with a protein like cheese. A suitable portion of fruit is a small one, such as a small apple, or cut a larger fruit in half. Stay away from canned fruit in heavy syrup and fruit juices and instead use fruit canned in it's own juices.

Don't be afraid of eating starches, but be sensible. Starchy foods turn into glucose in your digestive system so you don't want to overdo it. Breakfast is important but you may have to forgo refined cereals, fruit, and possibly milk in the morning if your sugars spike after this meal. If it does, you should have a breakfast of a protein in addition to a carbohydrate, like oatmeal, and see if that works better. Choose cereals with extra bran or fiber.

THE HASSLES OF COOKING AND EATING RIGHT

Many pregnant women with GD find it a real inconvenience when changing their eating habits. They are already restricted from taking most all medications (unless deemed necessary) and have cut out things like alcohol and caffeine. The planning is time-consuming. They feel punished more than anything when it comes to what they can put on their mouths. There are some helpful hints for cutting time and making up for what you can't have.

Issue #1: It is an inconvenience to cook two different meals for the family.

Solution: Everyone can eat the same meal; there is no need to make two meals all the time. Just prepare one meal but flavor it two different ways. Like on the night you have spaghetti, make a complex, bold-tasting sauce for the adults, but heat up jarred spaghetti sauce for the kids. When making casseroles, you can put the healthier recipe on one half of the dish and put the regular recipe on the other half. You can make a healthy burrito with a whole wheat tortilla, while everyone else uses a plain tortilla. You may get by serving a healthy meal without anyone noticing it. For example, when you make pumpkin muffins, your family will undoubtedly not realize that they are low-fat since the pumpkin makes them so moist.

Issue #2: It takes so much time to prepare healthy meals.
Solution: When you go to the store, choose frozen or fresh packages of precut vegetables and other healthy foods. This will help cut time in the kitchen. Also look for precut carrots, broccoli, cauliflower, and other vegetables sold in individual bags or tubs in the produce aisle. Lettuce is available like this and is also in kits where you can have a variety of salads at your disposal. Caesar salad, romaine lettuce, baby lettuce… there are so many to choose from! Many stores have salad bars as well, so you can choose from an array of vegetables and fruit. Just try to stay away from any that are covered with sauce. You can find in the meat department an assortment of marinated meats, rotisserie chicken, and fish prepped to take home and cook. Refrigerated reduced-fat dough, like from Pillsbury, make a great side for a meal. Low-fat cheeses are packaged and ready to go in the dairy section. Canned vegetables and fruit (in juice) are the way to go for easy meal preparation.

Issue #3: Healthy foods do not taste good.
Solution: Your health food should not taste bland! There are many herbs and spices that you can use that will not impact your blood sugar. Tape a chart of different herbs and spices that complement different dishes in your kitchen cupboard for easy reference. For instance, rosemary goes well with beef and thyme is great with chicken. Some people like lemon pepper for their fish. Garlic is healthy for you and goes with many dishes. Add to

your list sun-dried tomatoes, balsamic vinegar, salsa, and lemon juice.

Issue #4: We love to eat out!
Solution: Eating out is such a problem because, for one thing, you don't know what the restaurant puts in their food. It could be corn syrup added to the Mongolian Beef or a sauce on your noodles. It is recommended to limit eating out or having takeout meals to once or twice a week. Also you need to make smart and informed choices. Instead of creamy or fried food, order meals that are grilled, baked, or steamed. Ask for sauces to be put to the side so you can use them to dip your food into it lightly, where you can control the amount. If the meal is scanty on the vegetables, ask for extra. At dessert time, you can ask for fruit or sorbet. You don't need to feel that you are deprived.

Issue #5: Our family is used to eating convenience foods and ready-made meals.
Solution: There are many, many ready-made meals today. Most of them are very unhealthy, loaded with sodium and fat. You can find there are some made to be healthier versions of your favorite meals. This is when you need to start reading the nutritional labels.   Some of these "healthy" meals may just be the smaller version of the regular meal. All of them will have a label on back so you can work them into your plan. You can always them healthier by adding more vegetables. Always drain canned vegetables because they are full of sodium. Rinse them thoroughly to remove most of it. Not only do you get more to eat by adding vegetables, but you feel fuller longer.

Issue #6: It costs a lot of money to eat healthy.
Solution: Healthy eating is not as expensive as much of the processed foods you buy. A potato, for instance, has much more bulk and nutrition then a small bag of potato chips. Snack sizes

of potato chips costs much more than a single potato! When you eat more fruits and vegetables, you will be eating these in place of some of the expensive meat and processed food you won't be eating.

Issue #7: I don't think I can give up all of my favorite foods.

Solution: You shouldn't have to give up any of your favorite foods. You just have to know how much you can have. You can talk to your diabetes nurse or dietitian about how to incorporate your favorite foods in your meal planning. All it takes is a bit of knowing how much and when you can have it. If you want a cupcake, you have to count it as carb choices based on nutritional information. You will want to eat it at lunch or supper and save your other carb choices for something healthier. Now you can say you can have your cake and eat it too!

Issue #8: It is too hard to eat right around other people.

Solution: It is important to talk to your family and friends about the changes you need to make for the next couple of months. You need to explain to them it is for the good of the baby and for you. Ask them not to tempt you will foods you shouldn't eat or complain because they are not having treats as often. They can still have their treats but ask them to have them while out of the house. See if they will be willing to try some of the meals you prepare and tell them they can give their feedback on how it tastes, etc. Kids love to be asked for their input on things.

Issue #9: I will not enjoy all this healthy food. I will be miserable.

Solution: If you know what foods you cannot do without, you may be able to find a healthy substitute for it. If you crave chocolate, you can try a darker chocolate that is less in carbohydrates. If it's cake you love, see if you can enjoy it with sugar-free pudding for the frosting or whipped topping. You are doing it for the baby for a limited time.

Issue #10: I feel like I am being punished if I can't go out to eat once in a while.
Solution: You can go out to eat if you prepare yourself beforehand. If you are going to a friend's house to eat, you should eat a snack before you leave so that you have greater control over your eating. Food can be less tempting if you have already eaten a fulfilling snack. If you go to a restaurant, share your meal with a friend or choose the healthier selections on the menu. If the serving size is large, you can save the rest for a to-go container or order from the ala carte menu. Then you can enjoy the rest at a later time or share with your significant other.

Issue #11: I really hate dieting.
Solution: You are not on a diet! You are not trying to lose weight (unless recommended by your doctor). Meal planning is when you are trying to place your foods in the day where it benefits you nutritionally. You can space out an allotted amount of carbohydrate throughout each day so you can maintain healthy blood sugar levels. So, you are not trying to restrict the amount of food you eat as you are watching your carbs.

Issue #12: Sitting down to plan my meals seems to be a waste of time.
Solution: Once you develop a meal plan, the hard part is over. You will get to know what foods have what carbohydrate units in them. It is only for a couple of months that you need to plan out your meals. You just want to make sure you place your carbohydrates evenly throughout the day so that you don't experience any hypoglycemic episodes. Taking the time to plan will make you feel much better in the long run.

You can place your favorite foods in the plan so that you can enjoy them without the worry of raising your blood sugar, as long as you watch your portions and read labels.

WHAT TO KEEP IN YOUR NEW HEALTHIER KITCHEN

Pantry:

Canned beans

Canola and extra-virgin olive oil and cooking sprays.

Cereals high in fiber content

Fish, canned (tuna, salmon)

Grains, such as brown rice, barley, oats.

Low-carb whole-wheat bread, pancake mix, tortillas.

Low-fat popcorn (snack-size bags).

Low-fat whole-wheat crackers

Low-sodium canned tomatoes and soups

Reduced-sugar jams, jellies, pancake syrups

Whole-grain pasta

Peanut butter

Refrigerator:

Fresh lean protein:

> Beef

> Boneless skinless chicken breast

> Eggs

> Ground turkey white meat

> Meat-substitute/soy products.

> Pork tenderloin

Salmon

Tofu

Turkey breast

Fresh vegetables

Low-fat milk

Low-fat or fat-free cheese

Low-fat or fat-free yogurt

Low-fat salad dressings

Fresh fruits

Freezer:
Berries of different varieties

Frozen vegetables

Frozen stir fry kits

Frozen lean protein: fish (tilapia, salmon, etc.); egg substitutes; beef; chicken

They always say not to go to the grocery store on an empty stomach and this idea holds so true, especially when you are watching what you eat. Label reading will take some time with the grocery trip, but once you know what you can and can't have, it will get easier. Here is a handy checklist you can use to prepare for your grocery trips.

GROCERY SHOPPING LIST

Refrigerator

PROTEIN

Eggs or egg substitute

Meat (lower in fat is recommended)

STARCHES

Bagels

English muffins

Low-fat tortillas

VEGETABLES

Asparagus

Broccoli

Carrots

Celery

Corn

Cucumbers

Lettuce

Mushrooms

Onions

Peppers

Potatoes

Spinach

Squash

Zucchini

Tomatoes

FRUIT

Apples

Avocados

Berries

Bananas (small)

Cherries

Grapefruit

Grapes

Kiwi

Lemon

Melon

Oranges

Peaches

Nectarines

Pears

Plums

DAIRY
Low-fat cottage cheese

Fat-free or low-fat yogurt

Reduced-fat cheese

Skim or 1% milk

FATS
Margarine with plant sterols or contains Omega 3s are better

Freezer
Fish fillets or shellfish

Frozen chicken breast (boneless, skinless)

Frozen fruit

Frozen meals (lower-sodium, lean options)

Frozen vegetables

Fat-free or low-fat frozen yogurt

To Cook With
Olive oil

Seasonings containing no salt

Balsamic vinegar

Lemon juice

100% whole wheat bread or pita bread

Brown rice

Canned beans (low-sodium preferable)

Canned fruit (canned in juice)

Canned tuna, salmon, or chicken

Dried fruit

Fat-free refried beans

Instant oatmeal or quick oats (plain)

Natural peanut butter or another nut butter

Pasta (try whole wheat)

Popcorn (light, microwave)

Potatoes (white or sweet)

Salsa

Sunflower seeds

Spaghetti sauce

Tomato juice

Unsalted nuts

Whole grain cereal, like oats or bulgur

Pantry

MAKING YOUR RECIPES HEALTHIER

Converting your favorite recipes is easier than you think. You can also make them tasty where you won't know the difference. Splenda with 50% sugar is great for baking and it will cut the carbs in your baked goods significantly. You can also use other ingredients to make your recipes lower in sugar but still maintain the taste.

Sugar hides in everything that you buy at the supermarket. If you are able to make your own food, you can reduce the amount your food contains. Not to mention, you will know exactly what is in your food. If you can reduce the sugar in many of favorite foods, you will substantially lower the carbohydrates. That means you can eat a little more of it! Adding fiber is a bonus since it slows the release of the sugar into the body.

Whole wheat flour can replace half of the white flour in a recipe without changing the texture too much. You may try reducing the sugar in a recipe by 1/3 (or even ½) and see if it still tastes good. Honey and molasses are like sugar in the way they raise blood sugar levels, however, they are concentrated with sweetness. You should be able to cut back on these sweeteners without sacrificing taste.

One idea to cut back on sugar is to use one tablespoon of sugar for each cup of flour when making banana bread and quick breads. These breads are more nutritious with the added fruit or vegetables (zucchini, pumpkin) so you are consuming more nutrients by eating them instead of white bread. Raisins and chopped apples can be put in the mix to add extra fiber. Something to note: when you reduce sugar in the recipe, the breads may not brown as well so spray a little oil on top before baking to help with that. Oh, and don't take the sugar out of yeast breads. They need it for the yeast to grow and make the bread rise.

Splenda offers a product that uses a combination of its sweetener and sugar to make baked goods. If you use just Splenda, the result will be drier cookies and cakes so you may want to add a little sugar to the mix if you want to prevent that. Ingredients like cinnamon and vanilla are great for helping the baked goods taste better.

Try adding more fiber to meals to stave off blood sugar spikes after eating. For your tacos and other meat-laden meals, you can replace some of the meat with more beans to increase the fiber. Keep the skins on potatoes when you make potato salad for a boost in fiber as well. Oatmeal in meatloaf is another way to sneak in fiber by replacing crackers or breadcrumbs.

Restaurant Eating

When eating out, it can be a treat or a way to ruin your carefully controlled meal plan. If you don't plan ahead and make sure you know what you should eat, it will cause you to possibly over eat and not feel good later. And if your baby gets too much extra sugar, they may stay up all night doing somersaults!

So before you even leave the house, make sure you know what's on the menu and what you are going to eat! Go to the websites for the restaurant or fast food place and read the nutritional information the companies provide. In some cases, it's even easy to add your meal together and see what it will be, but you will be surprised how quickly things add up!

Fast Food

Many people use fast food as a means for a quick meal on the way home from work. They don't feel like fixing a meal when they get home and it is fast and effortless. However, most fast food is loaded with fat and carbohydrates and wreaks havoc on blood sugar if you are diabetic. Most popular fast food chains are recognizing that the public wants healthier choices so they are offering more healthy options. You see more fruits and vegetables offered along with their salad options. Yogurt and low-fat ice cream is available, too. It just takes resolve on your part to skip the French fries and sundaes and order the healthful choices.

You can go out to eat with family and friends and still enjoy food rather than sit with a diet cola while they are enjoying their hamburgers and shakes. Let's take a look at some typical fast food places.

BURGER JOINTS

You can still order a hamburger; just order a small one or the kid's meal size. A small burger contains about 31 grams of carbs or 2 carb choices; you can also opt for the grilled ranch wrap which has 25 carbohydrates. A four-piece chicken nugget portion is a good choice with 12 carbs as well as the grilled chicken salad at 10 carbs. You can share a small fry (2 carb choices) with someone so you still get some but won't be going over your carb count for the meal. A full package of apple slices has only four grams of carbohydrates so you can indulge freely with no worries. Stay away from condiments if you don't know the carbohydrate content. Sweet and sour sauce is an easy tip off, but other sauces may full of sugar or corn syrup.

Wendy's® restaurant offers up an array of options that offer variety to those who are sick of salad options. Grilled chicken go-wrap and their junior hamburger both come in at 25 grams of carbs where their 4-piece chicken nuggets are worth one carb choice. The restaurant boasts of delicious chili, and it is only 20 grams of carbohydrate in a small serving. If you add crackers, however, this will increase the carb count. It's best to choose kids meals and salads to stay within your limits, however, watch out for the carbohydrate in the salad dressings.

TACO BELL®

If your friends want to go to Taco Bell, you will be happy to know that you can have tacos. They are around 1 grams of carbohydrates, or 1 carb choice a piece. Black beans on the side as 1 carb choice will complement a meal of two tacos. All of the sauces are low in carbohydrate; however, don't use more than 2 packets with your meal so you stay within your carb count. Best options on the Taco Bell menu are:

1 carb choice per serving:

Fresco Crunchy Taco

Fresco Chicken Soft Taco

Fresco Grilled Steak Soft Taco

Fresco Soft Taco

Crunchy Taco

Soft Taco-Beef

Chicken Soft Taco

Doritos® Locos Taco

All of Taco Bell® salads are over 57 grams of carbohydrate, so stay clear of them. You can enjoy a couple of tacos for a meal without going over your carbohydrate count.

SUBWAY®

Sandwich restaurants such as Subway is a great for low-fat dieters, but you still have to be wary of what you can have without going over your carb limit for the meal. All of the sandwiches are over 3 carb choices, and we're talking about the 6-inch, not the foot-longs. Your best bet here is ordering one of their salads, which are between 1 to 2 carb choices. Kid meals are around 30 grams of carbohydrate so this is another better option. Steer clear of the sweet onion sauce and honey mustard. These sweet sauces add an extra carbohydrate choice when mixed in the salads.

If your local Subway offers breakfast sandwiches, choose the 3-inch flatbread choices without the omelet. These sandwiches contain around 21 carbohydrates per serving. The 6-inch subs and omelet sandwiches have twice the carbs. Subway offers soup that won't hurt your carbohydrate budget. Many are lower than 20 carbohydrates for an 8 ounce bowl.

KFC®

There is mostly chicken at this restaurant but you can eat it in several ways. Grilled chicken is on the menu now, so it is a low-carb option and very flavorful. But the Original Recipe isn't something to avoid. A drumstick has only 3 grams of carbohydrates and the other dark pieces are about 6-8 grams. The chicken breast is worth one carb choice. The bad side to KFC is the fat content. Keep this in mind when you indulge in their tasty poultry. Their sandwiches will be what get you in trouble when watching your carbs. One sandwich contains 52 grams of carbohydrates! Most of the other sandwiches are not much better. And their chicken pot pie is oh-so-good but packs in about 66 grams a pie. The side dishes are not too bad, fortunately. Green beans are offered, and you know you can eat a lot of those! Mashed potatoes, as an individual serving, is only 19 grams of carbs. Use caution with the biscuits as well, because they count as carbohydrate choices too!

Where fast food is getting on the bandwagon for healthier food choices, many "sit-down" dining establishments are still lagging behind. This does not mean that you cannot go to these restaurants without blowing your carbohydrate budget, but it does mean some planning in advance. Dining at popular restaurants is a challenge because they serve immense amounts of food; more than a person should eat at one sitting. One option is planning ahead to eat only a portion of it and then taking the rest home. You can also see if you and another person can share the meal. You both would save money and you will avoid the temptation of eating the leftovers later.

ITALIAN

You might think you will never be able to eat at an Italian restaurant until you have your baby. It is true that high carb foods are served there. Garlic bread, pasta, and not to mention the high-fat sauces and meats that are part of most of their dishes. It can be a diabetic nightmare to walk into a place like this. There are things you can partake in; however, you need to know ahead of time what you can indulge in. Pasta is not a bad thing, but you need to limit the portion. It shouldn't be the main part of your meal. You can order a soup that has pasta in it. Ensure that you are getting only a cup of pasta (45 grams of carbohydrate) and you will be fine. Grilled chicken or fish would be a great option, but you may want to ask the server not to bring bread sticks to the table. This will remove any temptation to munch on these while waiting for your meal. Having the soup of the day and a salad would be a meal in itself, especially if you have unlimited salad.

MEXICAN

Mexican food… it is a carbohydrate haven, with tortillas, refried beans, and Spanish rice as part of every dish. Much of the ethnic fare is fried as well. First of all, do not allow the chips to be on your table. Ask the server to take them away. If you have to have some, just take a handful (about 15 chips) and be done with it. The salsa is a good condiment to have since it has very little calories to worry about. Dishes to eat at a Mexican restaurant can include meat and cheese, beans (though refried beans are high in fat), a small amount of rice, vegetables, and corn tortillas that are not fried. Corn tortillas are lower in carbs than flour. Fajita meat can be eaten without the tortillas, saving you from eating extra carbohydrates. You can try a taco salad without the fried tortilla bowl, pork carnitas, and enchiladas without the cheese sauce. You will have to ask the waiter to hold some of the ingredients that have carbs in them. You are paying for the food; you should get what you ask for.

CHINESE

Food served at a Chinese restaurant can send your blood sugar to all-time highs if you are not careful with what you order. You wouldn't think it since most of the meals are comprised of vegetables and lean meat. However, the rice is one of the culprits to watch for. Egg rolls and sweet and sour sauce are guilty as well. You get a large portion of any of these carbs and your diabetes does not have a chance. Fortunately you can eat some of the dishes offered without worrying about your blood glucose reading later. Have yourself some hot and sour soup. Or try the wonton soup, which is also lower in carbs. Chop suey is another good dish to have. You can ask the server for less sauce on your meat and to increase the vegetables when you order stir fry. This way you cut back on any carbohydrates that may be lurking around in the sauce.

AMERICAN RESTAURANTS

There are some restaurants, like Applebee's®, that offer a section in the menu especially for dieters. You will also see nutritional information as well. If you can go to restaurants that offer more healthful choices, you will be more successful in staying within your goals. And don't forget that at restaurants like Panera Bread®, you can go online ahead of time and find out the nutritional information prior to going.

See if the meal you are considering has a lunch-size portion available. These tend to be a lot smaller portions than the ones offered at dinner. You may also order from the kids menu or senior plate, if the restaurant allows it. Choose low-carbohydrate vegetables to complement your meal. Baked and mashed potatoes add extra carbohydrates so if you have to have your potatoes, limit them by eating only ½ of a serving. Then consider it your starch for the meal.

Ask for a low-carb or no-carb dressing for your salad. Italian and Ranch dressings are lower in carbohydrates than French dressing, but all regular dressings are high in fat so you may want to have them offered on the side so you can control the portion. You may want to bring your own low-carb dressing in a small container just to be on the safe side. Stay away from croutons and fried chicken bits in your salad. Eating these may cause a rise in blood sugar.

If the waiter brings rolls to the table, you can have them sent back. You should avoid pasta dishes since the portions are large, unless you are sharing with another person. Many dishes have a starch in them like pasta, rice, and bread, so it would be best to stay with grilled meat, chicken, and fish instead. You will know you're not eating any hidden carbohydrates. Also, avoid anything fried and salty. Ask for fruit as your dessert so you don't feel deprived. The restaurant may even offer diet Jell-O.

You can plan to eat half of your meal and take the rest home to eat for leftovers. Consider eating soup and salad for your meal.

All it takes is a little time to plan your outing to a restaurant. Many of them offer nutritional information so that you can make an educated decision and stay on your eating plan. Remember you are diligently doing what is best for you and your baby for during the pregnancy.

Other Things You Should Know!

On the Road

When you and your family are traveling, there are many things to prepare for so you do not have trouble with low blood sugar or in the position of consuming more carbohydrates than you should. Here are some helpful ideas to consider before going out of town.

#1 -- Keep your supplies close at hand.

It is handier if you can keep your glucometer, insulin, and everything you need with you at all times, like in a purse you carry. If you pack everything away, you have more difficulty getting to it.

#2 – Try to stick to your routine.

It's all about staying on task with your meals, which can be a challenge when you are out of your routine. Try to eat every 3 hours and don't go any longer than that.

#3 -- Get documentation.

Make sure you have all of your health information documented in case of medical emergency, including your doctor's information and any special medications or allergies.

#4 -- Always be prepared to treat low glucose.

Ensure that you keep a close eye on your blood sugar and have a little candy or orange juice to consume if your sugar goes low.

#5 -- Investigate the food you eat.

You may want to plan ahead on restaurants where you will be eating and what types of food or drink you may come in contact with.

#6 -- Increase your stash of supplies.

It would behoove you to keep extra supplies handy to ensure you have what you need when you are out of town.

#7 -- Consider time zone changes.

Your schedule may need to be adjusted to accommodate the time zone changes.

#8 -- Test your blood sugar.

It is especially important to test your sugar when you are on vacation so that you monitor any fluctuations that may occur because of activity or new foods you are eating.

#9 -- Tell others that you have gestational diabetes.

It's a good idea to let others know you have GD just in case you have something happen, like pass out from a low blood sugar. Someone would be aware of your diagnosis and let the medical staff know so they can treat you appropriately.

When You Are Ill

There may be a time when you will become ill. You will not be able to keep food down and you may run a fever. If you are sick, your blood sugars will be higher since your body may be fighting off an infection. You should continue with your regular meal plan while increasing the intake of noncaloric beverages, like broth, water, and other decaffeinated beverages. You should also continue to take your diabetic medication and check your blood glucose every 4 hours. If it is higher than 240 mg/dl, let your health provider know.

When you eat less than normal, still continue the oral medication and/or insulin as prescribed. You will need to drink carbohydrate-containing fluids, such as soups, juices, and regular soft drinks (decaffeinated). This will help regulate your blood sugar while you are sick. If you cannot keep anything down, contact your doctor immediately. It is very important that you still keep taking your medications because of the liver's counter-regulatory mechanism. This is when the liver senses a drop in blood glucose and spills out much of its own glucose as a response, causing a high blood sugar. Food is important when ill though you do not want to eat anything. It is required so that the cells of your body have energy to deal with the stress of the illness. Extra insulin may be necessary to meet this demand.

So What Now?

Once you finish reading this book and put it down, you need to start with meal planning. Whether you choose counting carbs or "choosing your plate," pick one that works best for you and your lifestyle.

If you walk away knowing just one thing, let it be that you know how to read labels. This will be invaluable to you as you decide what foods to incorporate into your meal plan.

It is easy to forget that you need to check your blood glucose every day if not multiple times daily. You need to be diligent in keeping track so that you don't go back into your old eating habits. You can lie to yourself about what you put in your mouth, but the numbers will let you know if you strayed.

Let everyone know that you are serious about staying on target with controlling your gestational diabetes. Many people want to make sure a pregnant woman is fed well, but they are not usually educated on your nutritional needs with GD. Just politely refuse anything that doesn't go with your meal plan.

Lastly, you need your family for support. They need to know that you have to watch how much sweets and starchy foods you can have. There may not be the snacks they are used to around the house if you need to keep them out of the house due to cravings. You can encourage your children by telling them it is for the good of the baby.

AFTER PREGNANCY AND IN THE FUTURE

✓ Make sure to ask your doctor about testing for diabetes soon after delivery and again 6 weeks after delivery.

✓ Continue to eat healthy foods and exercise regularly.

✓ Have regular checkups and get your blood sugar checked by your doctor every 1 to 3 years.

✓ Talk with your doctor about your plans for more children before your next pregnancy.

✓ Watch your weight. Six to twelve months after your baby is born, your weight should be back down to what you weighed before you got pregnant. If you still weigh too much, work to lose 5% to 7% (10 to 14 pounds if you weigh 200 pounds) of your body weight.

✓ Plan to lose weight slowly. This will help you keep it off.

Eating healthy, losing weight and exercising regularly can help you delay or prevent Type 2 diabetes in the future. Talk with your doctor to learn more.

OTHER BOOKS IN THE GESTATIONAL DIABETES SERIES:

GESTATIONAL DIABETES DIET MEAL PLAN AND RECIPES: YOUR GUIDE TO CONTROLLING BLOOD SUGARS & WEIGHT GAIN (BABY STEPS FOR GESTATIONAL DIABETES) (VOLUME 1)

http://www.amazon.com/Gestational-Diabetes-Diet-Meal-Recipes/dp/0615747736/

GESTATIONAL DIABETES JOURNAL: KEEPING YOUR BABY HEALTHY (BABY STEPS FOR GESTATIONAL DIABETES) (VOLUME 2)

http://www.amazon.com/Gestational-Diabetes-Journal-Keeping-Healthy/dp/0615873928/

LIFE AFTER GESTATIONAL DIABETES: 14 WAYS TO REVERSE YOUR RISK OF TYPE 2 DIABETES (BABY STEPS FOR GESTATIONAL DIABETES)(VOLUME 5)

http://www.amazon.com/Life-After-Gestational-Diabetes-Reverse-ebook/dp/B00FZEGRXA/

Made in the USA
San Bernardino, CA
12 October 2018